Also by Jeff Hauswirth:

WHAT ARE YOU WAITING FOR? A Beginner's
Guide To Weight Training (Tate Publishing)

Now You Have No Excuses

Jeff Hauswirth

A.C.E. Certified Health Coach

Foreword by Dr. David Hill, D.C., C.C.S.P.

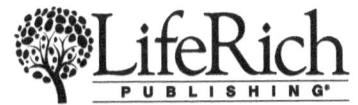

For more information, please check the following sites:
www.peacethroughstrengthfitness.com
www.advocare/com/13068922
www.facebook.com/WAYWF

LifeRich Publishing is a registered trademark of The Reader's Digest Association, Inc.

LifeRich Publishing books may be ordered through booksellers or by contacting:

LifeRich Publishing
1663 Liberty Drive
Bloomington, IN 47403
www.liferichpublishing.com
1 (888) 238-8637

Because of the dynamic nature of the Internet, any web addresses or links contained in this book may have changed since publication and may no longer be valid. The views expressed in this work are solely those of the author and do not necessarily reflect the views of the publisher, and the publisher hereby disclaims any responsibility for them.

Any people depicted in stock imagery provided by Thinkstock are models, and such images are being used for illustrative purposes only.
Certain stock imagery © Thinkstock.

ISBN: 978-1-4897-0290-6 (sc)
ISBN: 978-1-4897-0291-3 (e)

Printed in the United States of America.

LifeRich Publishing rev. date: 9/30/2014

Contents

Acknowledgements

First and foremost, I would like to thank my family and friends for always encouraging me and believing in me. I would not be where I am today without them. I would like to thank all those who have so far inspired me along my path. Without you, I would not be here. Thank you to the following people who are pictured in this book for not only being gracious enough to pose for this, but for also helping me design this work out and be my test group (listed in order of how they appear in the book): Ben Collaer (cover photo), Erin Hauswirth (my wife), Gunnar Stein, Austin Hill, my daughter, Megan Hauswirth, and Kyle LeClaire. Thank you also to Mrs. Tiffany Scullion for her editing expertise. Lastly, I would like to thank you, the reader of this book, for giving me a shot, and (hopefully) using the knowledge contained in this book to change your life.

I would like to dedicate this book to Hulk Hogan. I have never met him, but outside of my family, he was the one who, when I was a kid, got me on the path to "train hard, say my prayers, and eat my vitamins" and also to "believe in myself" as the 90's rolled upon us. I am still a proud Hulkamaniac, BROTHER!

Foreword

‒ ‒ ‒ ‒ ‒ ‒ ‒ ‒ ‒ ‒ ‒ ‒ ‒ ‒ ‒ ‒ ‒ ‒ ‒ ‒

The human body is designed to work and to exercise. The body needs exercise or it begins to break down. Weight training is a critical part of exercise and its benefits are obvious. However, I find many of my patients think a regular exercise program is overwhelming with their busy schedules or are downright intimidated to even start. Many think of themselves as non-athletes or that they are too heavy or weak to try or they just don't know what to do. Having a safe, simple, effective plan is critical to their short and long term success.

Jeff Hauswirth has done just that: he has developed a straight forward, easy-to-follow starter program which is effective for the novice as well as the conditioned athlete. Jeff has walked the walk as an athlete, a coach, and a teacher. Having gained years of practical experience and insight, <u>NOW YOU HAVE NO EXCUSES</u> cuts through the common blocks to exercise and breaks through common myths. His advice is good and his workout program is easy to follow.

I enjoy the routine myself. I have done the program with my 14 year old son. It works my whole body and I get it done in a short time. My son uses it for conditioning for skiing and finds it effective. My patients benefit because they have structure and guidance to a daunting task. I fully endorse Jeff's work and recommend it for my patients.

David Hill D.C., C.C.S.P.
Chiropractic Sports Physician

A Little on Me and
My Philosophy

- -

L ike many people, over the years I have had those thoughts of "some day, I will write a book about that." Well, I did. I was very excited about it (and still am). I owe a lot to Tate Publishing for taking a chance on me and offering to publish my book. My first book is called <u>WHAT ARE YOU WAITING FOR? An Introduction to Weight Training</u>. My first book is about how to get started into the world of exercise and weight lifting, and I highly recommend you buy that book if beginning to lift weights is something you want to do. It is a great guide to get you started (but I digress from what I want to tell you about).

Shortly after writing my first book, I started to think about those people who, for whatever reason, want to exercise, but don't have access to a gym. Or maybe, like some people I know, want to exercise, but are a bit self conscious about doing so in a place that is so public, like a gym. So, with those thoughts in mind, I am writing this book. I have created this workout to help you lose fat, gain muscle, boost your energy, and give you all the benefits of exercise, and it was created with the idea that it is something you could do in a prison cell (not that I am recommending you get incarcerated to do this workout, but my point is, you don't need a lot of space). As for equipment, at most, you will need a chair, a wall, and a mat. I do recommend getting some push-up bars, as well. I use them not only for added intensity, but also for wrist comfort.

Another thing I wanted to consider in writing this book was time. It seems that we have no "time" for things today. I really do not believe that is true. Years ago, I read a cartoon that summed the idea of time up. It went something like do you have time for 1 hour a day of exercise, or do you have time for 24 hours a day of being dead? It may sound extreme, but it is true. I know that there have been instances in my own life where I didn't have the time to do something and by and large (for most of us), that's a copout excuse. I think it is a copout because we have time for many other useless and menial things throughout our day (video games, television, web surfing, just to name a few), but it really comes down to priorities. Maybe you are a younger kid, and right now it seems more important to you to play on one of the many mind melting video consoles instead of be active, and you will worry about exercising and health when you get older. Here's a news flash: the habits you form as a youth will be those you keep as an adult. If you are young and lazy, what do you think are the odds that you will get motivated as you get older?

Maybe you are an adult with a job and kids, and you don't have that time. I am betting that somewhere in your day, you have time to take care of yourself. Personally, one motivating factor for me is that I do have kids. I want to be around a long time to watch them grow, and eventually watch them move on and have their own families so that I can spoil my grandchildren. Whatever your age, now is the time to stop making those excuses and start. If it makes you feel better, you could multi task while doing this program and put the television on. If you try and "find" the time for just about anything, you never will. If it means enough, you will *make* the time for it.

Personally, exercise has, in one way or another, been a part of my life since I was around the age of 14. I learned the importance of fitness my freshman year during my first training camp for high school football (for which, I was far from in shape enough to make a difference). I had begun weight lifting the summer before the season with my older brother, who was a college athlete. I should have taken it more seriously, and also participated in the running he did. To say that I lived and learned would be an understatement, but I did learn some valuable lessons.

Over the following 30 plus years since my introduction to exercise, I think I have learned a thing or two, and have shared these ideas with many friends and students. Through trial and error (and a lot of personal research), I have found out what works and what does not. I currently am a Middle School Physical Education/Health Teacher. I have been teaching for the better part of 17 years. I have my degree in Social Studies, Physical Education, and Psychology. I am also an American Council on Exercise (ACE) Health Coach. I love what I do, and I want to share with you some of my experiences to help you get moving.

Some things to consider here before you get started:

- First and foremost, make sure you are healthy enough for this (or any) type of exercise. It sounds strange I know, but there certain people who shouldn't do this. For your sake, make sure you are healthy enough (get a physical from your doctor).
- If this is your first workout routine, or if it has been a while for you since you have done any steady exercise, you will find that after the first day or two, your body will be mad at you. What I mean is that you will be sore. You might feel extra stiff in the morning when you wake up. Fight through this! Your mind will tell you that it is ok to just stop now, and never go back, but this is where you need to dig deep and find (develop) that mental toughness to work through it. You may even find that you actually wind up doing fewer repetitions your second or third time through the routine (like less on Thursday and Friday then on Monday and Tuesday). That's ok, and is no reason to quit! After the first couple of weeks, your body will start to agree with you about working out, and that initial soreness will go away. Start slow, and work up to what you want to be. As I learned long ago, you won't move mountains right away, but over time, you'll at least give them a good push.
- Never skip the warm up or cool down! These are designed to get the muscles ready for work, and then at the end help get them in a state of recovery. You are looking to risk injury should you skip these.

- Once you start, commit to it. What I mean is, if you only do this once or twice a week, you will not benefit from it, and it will frustrate you, and you will most likely quit, and then you will want to blame me because this plan "didn't work" for you. Well, as much as I would love to, I can't be there to help motivate you every day to put in the work. That has to come from within you. I will be there in spirit, though, if that helps. Try to find the same time every day to dedicate to putting the work in. If you use the same time each day, it will be easier to form as a habit.

- Work at your own pace. My intention for this plan is that you get each routine done, 3-4 times through, taking a 1 minute break after each 12 routine circuit. I don't expect you to start by getting that many sets in right away. I will (later in this book) explain how to ease into it. Getting started is the first step. You will find that once you do get started, you may need more breaks, or you might only be able to get through one series without stopping for the first few weeks. Or maybe you can't work for a whole minute. That's fine. Over time, you will get better, and over time, you can increase your work load. Whatever you got, give your all.

- Remember to breathe! It sounds funny, but I have actually seen people who "forget" to breathe, or purposely hold their breath, thinking it gives them some sort of edge. It doesn't, and it won't do you any good to hold your breath (unless you think passing out or maybe popping capillaries in your face is good). For the most part, inhale down, and exhale yourself back to the starting position for these moves. Once you get started, you will understand what I mean.

- It's not just about working out. It is also about what you eat, when you eat, and getting enough rest for your body to recover. You will find more information about this in the next chapter.

- If it helps, find a workout buddy and do this together. If you are one of those who are self conscious about working out with others, then of course you can go solo, but working out with a partner can also benefit you because you have someone to help motivate you and push you to keep working. I have found over the years that having a lifting or exercise partner also helps me stay disciplined to make sure I work out, because if I don't work out, then I may be letting them down.

- Lastly, if you want to see certain proof of change, about every 6 weeks (starting with the first day you start this exercise routine), take a frontal picture and a side shot of yourself to see how you change over time. I know how it can feel frustrating because we all want to change *right now*, but it doesn't work that way. You will not, I am sure, "feel" the change. You will notice things like "gee, these pants are a lot looser", or "wow, that feels pretty light", which is great, but one thing that will help keep you going forward is to see where you were.

This program has some stuff in it I am sure you have at least heard of, and maybe some you have not. Either way, I have created this program to work your whole body through a 4 day exercise routine. So, you have just a little bit of time left to sit back and relax as you read this book, but I do expect you to get up and start working. As I said before, now you will have no more excuses!

How to Fuel the Furnace

- -

One thing that seems to frustrate people is that it's not just exercise that makes a change. It is a combination of exercise, diet, and rest that makes a difference. When I say the word diet, I don't mean some sort of "lose 10 pounds in 3 days" type of thing. First and foremost, *those* types of diets rarely if ever work. Why? Well, you may lose weight, but your habits don't change. So, eventually, diets of this sort are bound to end, and if your eating habits haven't changed, you will bounce right back into the habits you had, and the weight will come right back. This is what many call the Yo-Yo Effect.

What I am talking about is your diet, meaning what you choose to put down the hatch on a regular basis. For better or worse, diet (according to some studies) is as much as 65% of a person's health! Let me say that again: SIXTY FIVE PERCENT! If you just do the workout and don't eat right, guess what? You are most likely wasting your time. It all flows together.

Do you want to do a little experiment? I tried this once, and it blew my mind. I had slowed my exercise down for one reason or another (I don't remember why), and, as you would expect, I started to add a few pounds to my frame. I went to the doctors for something completely unrelated, and I asked him about my weight. He, of course, asked about my diet, and I told him it was a healthy diet, with just the right amount of calories.

My doctor suggested that I write down everything I eat over a 3-4 day period. Then I could see if it was really enough or too much and if it was really healthy or not. Wow. That's about all I can say. I really learned something that day, and am very appreciative to my doctor for some simple advice. Give it a try. Write down everything you take in over a 3 or 4 day period, and see how you do. Be honest with yourself. If you put it in, write it down, and then after about 3-4 days, see how "healthy" your choices are. You may be as amazed as I was.

So what are the "right" choices? Most of us know what is good for us, but check your cupboards and see what's in there. I will wait. What did you find? My guess is at least some of it probably could be better for you. Most of us, even with all the knowledge that is available on what to eat, how much to eat, and all that other stuff, still make choices that lack health, because it is easier to just grab and go then to take a few minutes to make sure it's good for us. It is much easier to be unhealthy in our society, because it is quicker. In reality, it doesn't take that much more time to find the good for you stuff.

For specific and detailed explanations on how much and what to eat, I highly recommend the web site www.choosemyplate.gov. This site replaces the mypyramid.gov site, and is a little easier to navigate.

Here are some general rule of thumb guidelines for eating, although I would really recommend you do some surfing around and check it out for yourself as well.

Drink water. Your body needs a minimum of half your body weight in ounces every day. So, if you are 150 pounds, you will need a minimum of 75 ounces of water each day to stay properly hydrated. That's for the "average" person. If you are in an environment where it is hot, or you have done a *lot* of intense work, you will need more. Consider the fact that your body is somewhere between 70-90% water, depending on what organ you are talking about (your brain is between 70-80% water, and your lungs, by some accounts, up to 90% water). So, how important do you think it is to make sure you get at least the daily recommended amount? Yes, you got it, very. One way to increase energy is to increase your intake of water (notice I am saying water here, not liquids like coffee, caffeinated drinks, etc.). Also, water can help with weight loss. For those of you who don't drink a lot of water, your body holds onto as much of it as it can. Increasing your water intake helps flush your cells, which will help with weight loss.

That whole thing about fruits and vegetables? Yeah, you need them. Depending on where you look, you should get somewhere between 5-13 servings a day (13? Really?). I personally shoot for 6-8 servings a day, but that is me. You can find out what is right for you by doing some personal research (or checking the above site). As far as fruits and veggies go, choose them in this order: 1 – Fresh, 2- Frozen, 3 – Canned. As much as you can, try and stay away from the juice type of servings. Even the 100% types of fruits and vegetables have things like sodium added to help preserve them. Especially watch out for fruit juices, as many companies add *way* too much sugar to make them more flavorful. If you do use canned veggies, rinse them well before heating to get as much of the preservatives off as possible.

Dairy is also a much needed part of your overall health. You should get 2-3 servings of dairy per day. Dairy products are usually high energy giving products, and include milk and milk products such as cheese and yogurt. There is this myth that dairy products are all high in fat. This really isn't true. Skim milk contains no fat. Many yogurts are also reduced or fat free. As for cheese, white cheese (like Mozzarella and so forth) are by and large lower in fat than yellow. Dairy products contain an excellent source of protein called whey protein (amongst other types, but you may have heard of whey). You can buy whey in pretty much every health store. One of the benefits of whey (other than its excellent protein) is that it naturally contains the branch chain amino acids (BCAA's), which are necessary for muscle growth. Don't skip the dairy! Dairy also contains a healthy dose of calcium which is good not only for bone strength, but is also being linked to weight loss, as well.

Another needed source of fuel comes from meats and protein rich foods (other than dairy). When most people think of healthy proteins, they automatically think of something like chicken and fish. Yes, excellent choices (as long as they are lean portions), but did you realize that certain beans (like soy or garbanzo beans) are also great sources? Eggs are also a great source of protein. Things like peanuts or (my favorite) almonds? Yup. Getting protein from nuts gives you another great supplement of your fatty acids (many fish are also high in this essential source). Fatty acids are linked to many thigns such as brain and heart health, along with fat loss. Lean cuts of beef and pork can also fit the protein bill. Proteins are extremely necessary for those who are exercising. Proteins contain amino acids (as mentioned in the dairy brief above). Amino acids are considered the building block of muscle. Hence, if you wish to build muscle, you need the proper bricks, so to speak. Your goal is somewhere between 5-7 servings per day.

Lastly, as far as what you eat, I get questions from a lot of people about supplements, and which are the "best" to take. Personally, I stick to the all natural stuff. I think I have tried about everything one can buy. I have stopped looking though, as I was turned on to Advocare health products. Advocare is a solid health and fitness company that has been around for 20 plus years. It has lots of non paid endorsers, and Drew Brees is their national spokesperson. Everything they make is basically as pure as it can be. They have an advisor team made up of literally hundreds of people from all forms of the fitness world (such as pro strength and conditioning coaches, college professors, etc.). Their Scientific and Medical Advisory Board has over 270 combined years! After many, many years of "break through" and "massive pumps" and "best ever" type of advertising, I have learned to go with the science, and for my money, Advocare wins, hands down. Want to learn more? Check out www.advocare.com/13068922. Yes, it is my Advocare site. I love their products enough that I also distribute them!

As I mentioned in the beginning, I work in a middle school. One *huge* mistake I see from kids (and many adults) is they don't understand what a true serving is. Look at your hand. Open it up, but keep your fingers and thumb as together as possible. See your palm? Imagine that your fingers are (for this visual) gone. That's approximately one serving of meat. Think about the last time you went out to a restaurant or cooked at home or the last time you had a piece of meat. Was it maybe a little bigger than your palm? I would bet it was a lot bigger.

With that same hand, imagine you are about to box, and make a fist. See how big that is? That is also a serving (of pretty much everything else besides meat). Think of the last time you went out. Do you think whatever was on your plate fit that description? My guess is probably no. Take a minute and mull over that thought. All those extra calories.

They have to go somewhere, right? Your body does eliminate some of it, but a lot of it is also stored for later use as fat.

It starts to make sense about why we as a society overeat. Many of us see the one thing placed in front of us and think "well, that must be my serving". Think about something as simple as a 20-ounce bottle of soda pop. One bottle, one serving, right? Um, no. Read the label. Odds are, there are 2.5 servings in that bottle. Even the "healthy" drinks like certain flavored waters can be misleading. Many of us see one little bottle, so it must be only one serving. Nope. Not even close. 2.5 total servings in that small 20-ounce bottle. Now, let's look at the nutritional value. Take the amount of carbohydrates in that bottle per serving (carbohydrates is basically another word for sugar). Multiply that amount by 2.5, because most of us will drink the whole bottle in one sitting. That number is how much sugar you are getting at one time. It is easy to do, and I am not saying that companies are deliberately misleading people or doing anything wrong, because they put it all on the nutrition label. But, really, how often do you read that? Ok, so now my point. If you don't already, start reading the label! Roughly, for about every 4 grams of sugar, there is one teaspoon. All those added calories. Your body stores extra carbohydrates as what? Yup, fat. Does that make carbohydrates *bad* for you? No, but too many, or those from empty calorie sources can be. Think of empty calories as those calories you take in, but they do little to nothing to fill you up or give you anything in the way of nutrition.

Along with this workout, which we will get into in a bit, another great way to help boost your metabolism is to get away from eating three big meals a day. Science has found that our bodies burn more efficiently when we eat 5-6 smaller meals a day. Think about it. If you are constantly fueling the fire, your metabolism has to keep churning to help digest food. Eating those three big meals a day will speed it up for a bit, but then sort of slow it down to a normal rate. Also, the three big meals a day can cause you to feel hungrier between meals. After eating, your blood sugar level jumps way up. To counter this (and to help deliver the energy where it needs to go), your body dumps a massive amount of insulin into your system, so you get this spike of insulin. Ever notice how after a bigger meal you feel a little sleepy? This is caused by the insulin spike. It jumps up for somewhere between 2-2 ½ hours after a meal, and then will return to a more normal level. This spiking, as it is known, leads to that sleepiness, and can also lead to feelings of hunger, which can lead to more snacking to satisfy that feeling.

If you are eating every 2-3 hours or so, your metabolism has to keep up with the digesting. Eating smaller meals more often throughout the day has also been proven to keep insulin levels more regulated, and help with keeping that "oh, am I hungry!" feeling to a minimum, hence, helping to avoid the binging. If you need to read that again, please do. It does sound a bit confusing at first. I would also recommend you do your own research, to confirm what I am saying.

But wait a minute, 5-6 times a day? How in the world will I have time for this? I hear you now. It is possible. You don't have to stop everything and cook up a meal every two hours. There are many companies that make excellent snack bars full of all the goodness of the proper vitamins, minerals, carbohydrates and proteins you need to get you through. There are even replacement drinks you can use, as well. Also, in between meal times is a great way to make sure you are getting your fruits and vegetables. It is not that difficult to munch on an apple or an orange, or have some carrots, is it? You may find that it does take a little more time to plan and prepare what and when you are going to eat, but, on the whole, the time spent doing this will more than be beneficial for you. It will also give you the opportunity to actually think about what you are eating. Honestly, in this grab and go world, how often do we actually think about what we put in the furnace?

You might be thinking that, after reading the above material, if you do veer off the healthy stuff, you will be eternally banished. Here's where I might get a bit hypocritical, but bear with me. It is ok to have things that may not be totally good for you (that's a nice way of saying junk food). *However*, moderation is the key! We are designed to eat what tastes good, right? If not, why do we have taste buds on our tongue? If you were to never have any of the "treats" in life, you might one day explode into a binging fury that lasts for months!

It is ok to occasionally reward yourself. One example that I like is that I pick one day a week (for me it is Sunday). If I have had a good week as far as eating right and exercising, I will reward myself with having a cheat meal or two on Sunday. This is my day to work for, because I love things like pizza, tacos, and chocolate. Now, this *one day* of veering off won't ruin me, and I still make sure to get my fruits and veggies, along with my needed water for the day. Eating like this every day? *Bad idea!* That's where the moderation comes in to play. Now, if I didn't have such a good week, I have to "punish" myself by sticking with the normal eating routine. Trust me, that doesn't happen often, because I love Sundays.

Maybe you don't want to do it like that, and that's ok. Maybe you are one who occasionally, throughout the week, like to have a treat. Go for it! Remember; keep it in perspective and moderation. Maybe you don't need that treat every day, right? Maybe you don't need that reward 2-3 times a day. When it comes down to it, you now (if not before) should have a basic grasp of what is right and what is wrong for you as far as keeping your fire going at a healthy level. The choice ultimately comes down to what you want to get out of this workout and your life.

So, the last piece of this total package is getting the proper rest. If you just exercise, or if you just eat right, you won't be optimizing what you could be getting. To me, health and fitness is a three pronged attack. Missing any of the three is cutting the efficiency of the others. You (we) need a minimum of 7-9 hours of sleep each day, depending on age and so forth. Obviously, for most of us, this happens at night. When you sleep, your body releases hormones that help you grow and recover. It is your body's natural way of supplementing, if you will. Shorting yourself with rest is shorting your workout, and will also lead to sluggishness, which can make it easier to skip workouts, and maybe even make it easier to eat those high sugar foods to get the boost of energy you desire. Don't short yourself. All three of these phases (exercise, diet, and sleep) are equally important to making you more efficient.

Laying Out A Plan

- -

S o, you bought this book, and I thank you. Now, think for a minute. Why did you buy this book? I think you made a great choice, but what do you want to get out of this? One road block that some find when beginning a program is that they really don't know where they want to go. That gets frustrating, so they stop and get nothing out of it, which leads to more frustration. I don't want that to happen to you, so bear with me here for this chapter.

At the end of this book, you will find a weekly workout sheet, which I highly recommend you use. On this workout sheet there is an area for you to write down a weekly goal, along with daily goals. As you get started, I would strongly encourage you to fill in both sections, to get you thinking about what you want. In a sense, having a goal is like laying out a blue print. I don't think you would build a house without a plan, would you? So, don't remodel yourself without knowing what you want.

Earlier, I had mentioned taking pictures about every 6 weeks to get a sense of how you are changing. You can also use that 6 week period to have a long term goal in mind, as well. You can think of the daily and weekly goals as your short term goals, and the 6 week goal as your long term goal. Of course, you can shorten or lengthen your long term goal, it's up to you.

When you think about what you want, make sure whether it is short term, long term, or whatever, that your goal fits two criteria: (1), that it is achievable (realistic), and (2) you can measure it. These are must haves for any goal you set, whether (in my opinion) it is for exercise or life. If it is something you can never reach, or something you don't really know if you have met, odds are you will get frustrated and quit.

So how will you know if it is realistic? That should be easy, but here is an example. Let's say you are just starting out with this program. Something realistic and measurable might be that you want to get your workout in by 8pm every day. Is that realistic? Can you tell when you have accomplished this? Yes and yes. Stay away from words like better, or more. They are too hard to really measure.

Now, let's say that you set some goals (or at least one), and you know they are realistic and measurable, and you begin to stride toward them, but for one reason or another you don't reach that goal. Does this make you a failure? Uh, *no!* This, by no means, should be a message for you to quit. Maybe you set your goal a little too high (possible). How close did you get to achieving it? Maybe you didn't allot enough time to accomplish it. Re-evaluate, reset, and keep working.

Along with goal setting, to challenge yourself throughout this program, set a goal in your head for each move. If you accomplish it, great, keep going if there is time and you feel up to it, or stop here and catch your breath for a second while the time finishes. If you don't accomplish it, write down what you did, so you can re-evaluate for the next time you hit this move.

Speaking of the worksheets, save them. It is also another great way to measure where you were and where you are, which will ultimately help you figure out where you can go. Along those lines, after each move, take 5 seconds to record your results. Don't expect to remember what you did at the end of your workout for each move. The combination of work and stress to your body will most likely not allow you to remember.

The Workout

- -

I hope you didn't skip all the stuff before this to get started. If you did, then you should really turn back to the beginning and get the basis for this routine. First and foremost, before I get into the movements, I want to make clear: *quality is way more important than quantity!* You will get a ton more benefit out of doing each rep perfect than you will if you are trying to get through as many as possible in the allotted time. Do not sacrifice form for numbers, ok?

This workout is a 4-day program, and ultimately, should take you less than an hour to finish. If it is taking you longer, you need to turn up the intensity a little. I call this a flip workout, because each week you will flip where you start. It will make sense in a minute, I promise.

For the first week, you will do the upper/abs workout on Monday and Thursday. On Tuesday and Friday of the first week, you will do the lower workout. For week two, you will flip this, and do the lower on Monday and Thursday, and the upper/abs on Tuesday and Friday. Pretty simple, hey? Wednesday, Saturday, and Sunday could be used for things like light cardio, stretching, and maybe pick one of those days to be a designated off-day. Whatever your choice, stick to the diet plan (unless it is your cheat day). No matter how hard you work, you will never out work a bad diet.

Ultimately, each exercise should be done for one minute, and do as many as you can with proper form during this minute. Along with this, you should be doing 3-4 sets (meaning go through each exercise in order 3-4 times per workout). I highly recommend that, if you are just starting an exercise program, or have been away from working out for a while, you should cut the time down to 30 seconds to start, and keep your sets to no more than 2. As you feel more comfortable and confident, slowly begin to add time to each exercise. Time first, then sets. An example of this could be go from 2 sets of 30 seconds each to 2 sets of 45 seconds each. Then 3 sets of 45 seconds each. You can decide what is best for you, but, the ultimate goal is 3-4 sets, 1 minute each.

So set a number goal that you plan to work toward in a specific time. That sounds a bit confusing. Let's look at this a little bit. Let's say you pick a goal of (for whatever exercise) 25. As the time ticks away you reach 25, but still have time left. It is perfectly fine to work past your goal, should you choose. If you want to stop here to catch your breath a little, that is ok, too. For some of these moves (the 3-stage push-up comes to mind) you will have to modify the time versus number idea. Since there are 3 different types of push-ups, you could do (let's say) 20 seconds of each style, or just do a certain number for each style. Your choice. Work to make each repetition perfect. Keep in mind through every move that form over speed is what you need. Remember: do as many as you can with good form, *not* just as many as you can.

As mentioned before, after each 12 circuit cycle, take a 1-minute break. In the beginning, you may need more or longer breaks. Challenge yourself, but as I said before, keep it attainable. This program is also designed to give you a cardio benefit as well, so push yourself through as much as your ability will allow. You will get tired, and that's ok. That is where you get the cardio benefit along with the muscle growth benefit. As you continue, you will see that you get benefits of both cardio activity plus resistance training. It's a beautiful thing!

I will explain each move shortly, but for now, here are the moves for each category:

Upper/Abs	*Lower*
3-stage push-up	Hindu Squat
Horizontal Side Knee Lift	1-leg Dead Lift
A-Frame Push-up	Back Bends
Side to Side Plank	Flutter Kicks
Side Shuffle	Wall Sits
Inch Worm	Tip Toe Leans
Chair Dip	Plyo-Jump
Whacky Jack	Sneaky Lunge
Twist Wrist Push-up	Alternating Knee Bends
Decline Push-up	Mule Kick
Dive Bomber	Side Hops
Horizontal Pull-up	Mountain Climber

As mentioned earlier, before you jump into whatever workout it is for that day, you need to warm up and stretch properly. A good warm up starts with getting the blood flowing through any number of choices. Things to help with this would be running in place for 2 minutes, doing some jumping jacks (50-100 would be a good start), or maybe combining these. It is important to get your muscles warm before stretching. A muscle is more pliable (stretchy) when it is warm, and that means reducing the risk of injury. As for the cool down, you should go through the stretches that you did in the beginning to help your muscles begin to recover.

Go through each of these stretches at least twice before you start to exercise, taking a few seconds between each to allow your muscles to recoup a bit. The proper form starts here, with the stretching. It's not about whipping through the tretching to get started. Take your warm up and cool down seriously to help reduce/avoid the risk of injury. In all, the warm up and stretch should take you around 3-5 minutes to complete. It's very important, so don't skip it. I can' stress that enough!

Upper/Abs Stretches

Here are some stretches you should do before and after each workout:

Start with your feet shoulder width apart, back straight, head looking forward, shoulders relaxed and fingers pointed to the floor (from here on out, we will consider this the base stance). Inhale. As you exhale, lean your head to the right so that your ear touches (or attempts to) your shoulder. Once you have completed the exhale, slowly inhale and raise your head up. Exhale and lean to the other side. Perform this 2-3 times per side. (Neck Stretch)

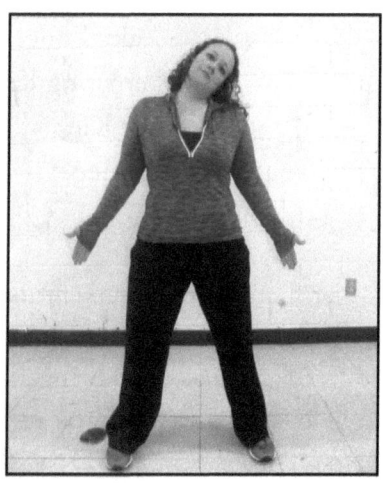

Stand facing a wall and raise one arm up so that it is parallel with the floor. Place your arm against the wall so that it is completely flat, and so that your chest is touching the wall. Slowly rotate your body away from your outstretched arm, but make sure that your arm stays parallel with the floor. Hold this for 10-30 seconds. Repeat this stretch on the other arm. (Wall Stretch)

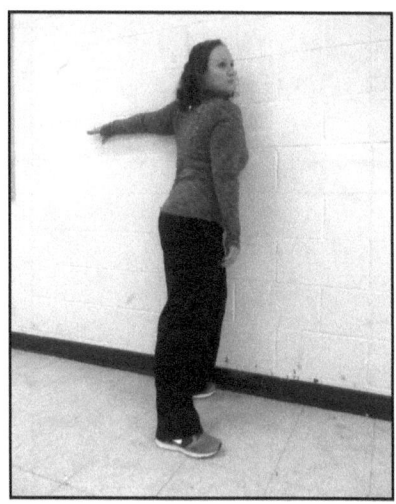

From the base stance, take one arm and place it across your body, just under your chin. With your other arm, hook the upper part of your arm and gently pull. Hold for about 10-30 seconds. Repeat this move on the other arm. (Static Hugger)

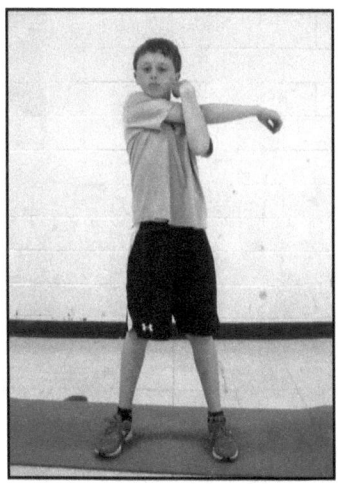

Take one arm and extend it above your head. Bend the elbow behind your head, and grasp either your wrist or elbow (if you are that flexible) and pull your arm until you feel the stretch in your triceps. Hold for 10-30 seconds. Repeat on the other arm. (Overhead Bent Arm)

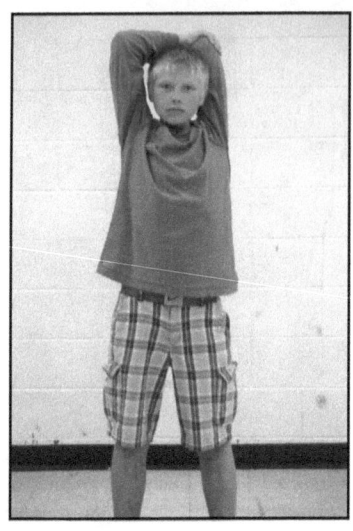

Put your arms straight down in front of you, and cross your wrists, placing the palms together. Try to roll the shoulders to touch in the front. Hold for about 10-30 seconds. (Straight Arm Clasp)

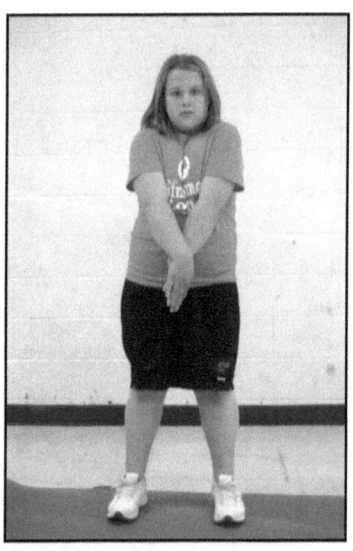

Clasp your hands behind you, elbows bent (to start) in the small of your back. Straighten your arms and roll your shoulders back so that you stand up straight, chest out, as if you are trying to touch your shoulder blades together. (Reverse Straight Arm Clasp)

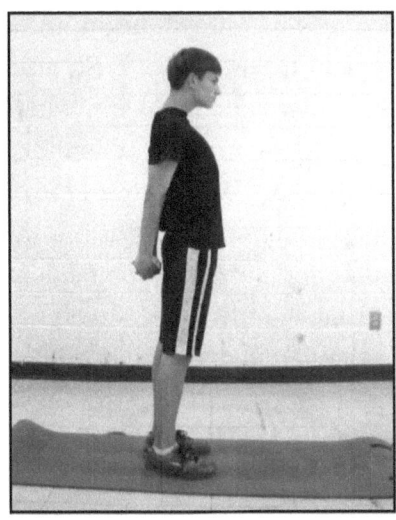

Lay flat out on your belly, hands up near your shoulders. Press your upper half up into the air, while keeping your hips on the ground. Gently look up, as if you are trying to sneak a peek behind you. If you can't get your arms totally straight before your hips come up too far, then get your arms as straight as possible. Hold for 10-30 seconds. (Cobra Stretch)

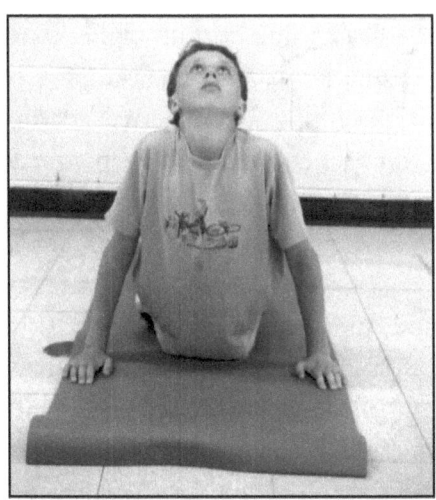

Upper/Abs Workout

21

For many of these moves, you will begin in the push-up position. I want to explain the right form for this. First, unless otherwise noted, your hands should be under your shoulders, with your arms straight. Be mindful that your back is straight (it sounds funny, but it helps to squeeze your butt together). As for your head, keep it in a neutral position, not looking up, and not looking at your feet. Also, be wary of your mid section, and keep tightness in your abdominal area. This may be something to experiment with. There are no sit-ups in this routine, but holding your abs tight and back straight will give them a workout. If you squeeze too tightly, you will be too stiff for some of these moves. From here on out, I will refer to this position as the starting point.

For many of these, I recommend push-up bars for at least wrist comfort if not also increasing your range of motion. I will put this beside the exercises I would use them in the explanation section. As for your movements, for the most part (if it varies from this, I will explain when necessary) your feet should stay steady and in one spot (no rocking them back and forth). Your hands should also stay locked in position, and your whole body should stay in position as you move up and down. Many people when doing any sort of plank or push-up routine, develop a habit of having a sway back, in which the belly hits the ground with the head being held up higher than the mid section. Another common error is known as going camping, in which a person's butt will poke up in the air like a tent. As you get started, be conscious of your position. The proper form is to keep your legs straight, back straight, butt tight, abs flexed. Everything between your hands and toes should move down and up as one. Very much like a 2x4 piece of lumber. As for depth, bring your body down as far as you can without touching the ground, then return to the start position.

You may find that early on you can't get all the way down and up again. That's fine. Go as deep as you can to maintain good form, and as time goes on you can work on depth. I also think it is ok (if you need to) to drop your knees to the ground if you find some of these difficult. Over time you will improve (provided you stay committed to working out), and you will eventually rise up to the more traditional position. I realize there is a stigma to doing push-ups on one's knees. I will not lie to you. I have at times dropped to my knees in order to finish a set. Should you be in this category, make sure the rest of your form stays as we discussed.

3-Stage Push-ups (push- up bars)

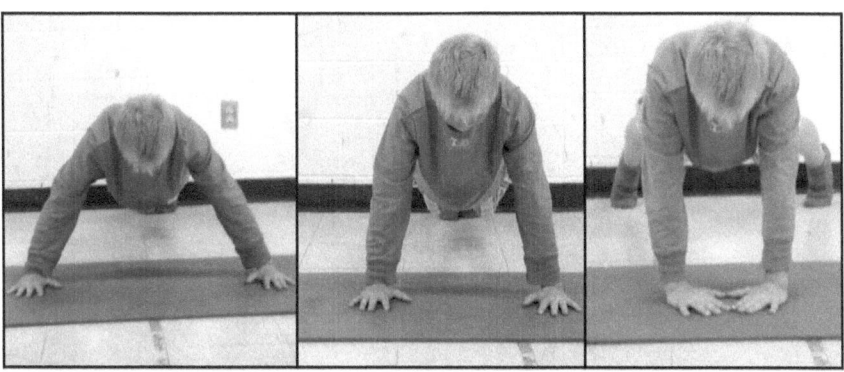

If you are doing this routine by timing each exercise, then divide the time by 3 (so if you are planning to go for one minute, you will go 20 seconds for each stage of this move). If you are doing it for a set number, work to get the same number per stage. For the most part, you will remain in the start position. The only variation is that your hand width will be moving. All else stays the same. Begin with your hands wider than your shoulders. If you choose to use push-up bars, be careful not to get too wide, as you will wind up pushing out instead of down and the bars could slip and cause injury. A good distance for width would be to look where your hands are placed in the normal starting point. Now, slide your hands out so that your thumbs line up where your pinkies were. Stick in that range, or maybe a touch wider. Starting with the wide hands, begin. Once you have finished the wide hand version, immediately slide your hands in to the starting point position and continue. Once you have finished, bring your hands close enough together so that your thumb and index fingers touch to form a diamond shape, and continue. For this 3rd and final stage, the object is to lower your chest down to where it slightly touches the diamond shape you have created. As you go down, keep your elbows tight to your sides.

They should rub your ribs as you go down and up. If necessary, it is ok to drop to your knees to keep this exercise going. If you have never done a diamond push-up, you will see what I am talking about the first time you give this move a whirl. Lastly, if you are using push-up bars, when you get to the diamond push-ups don't use the bars.

Horizontal Side knee Lift (push-up bars)

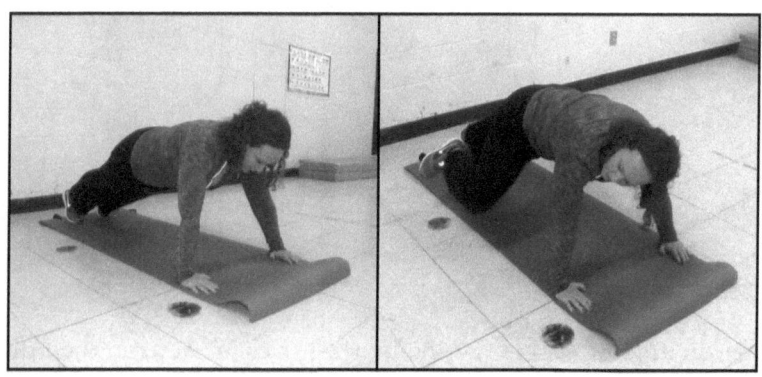

From the Starting point, bring your left knee up towards your elbow, while at the same time, rotating your leg out. As your knee comes forward, look back toward your foot. This will help you bring it up closer to your elbow. Slowly guide it back to the starting position, and repeat the same move with the other leg. As for doing repetitions, let's say you do 5 on each leg. That only counts as 5 reps, *not* 10!

A-Frame Push-up (push-up bars)

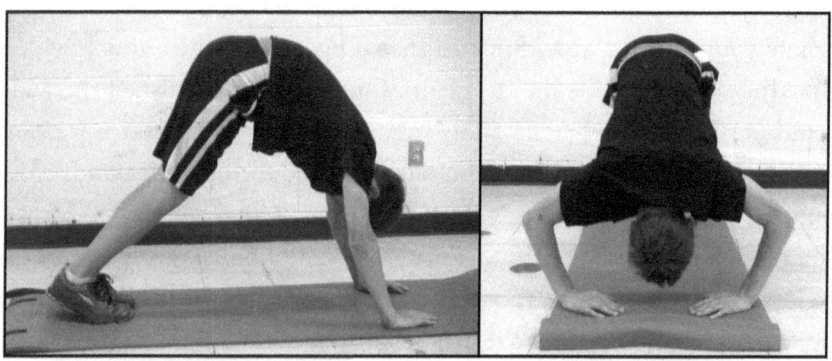

To get the right form, get into the starting point, and place your hands as if you were going to do a wide push-up. From here, walk your feet in toward your hands as far as you can, but make sure your legs stay straight and your feet stay together. From this position, bend your elbows and lower your body down toward the ground as if you are trying to touch the very top of your head to the ground (*not* your face!). Make sure that your legs stay straight. Push back up to straighten your arms. Down and up is one repetition. If you have never done this before, I will caution you that it is difficult, as this move isolates your shoulders. As you gain confidence in this, to challenge yourself you can use the push-up bars. If you feel supersonic, use the push-up bars and also place your feet up on a chair, but make sure that your backside remains higher than your feet.

Side to Side Plank

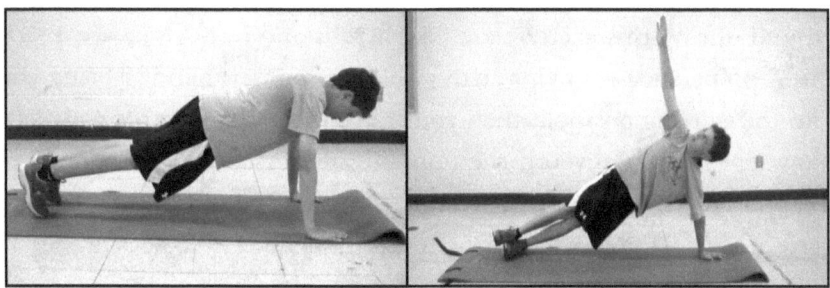

From the starting point, rotate your body to the side. Make sure you get a good base with your feet (place one on top of the other). As you rotate, the only part of you that should be touching the ground is the side of one foot and your hand. Your opposite hand should be as straight up as you can get it, sort of making your body a sideways "T". Do not allow your body to slack or sag. Keep everything from your arm pit to your ankle stiff like a 2x4. Once you accomplish this move on one side, slowly return to the starting point and rotate to the other side. Again, one rep equals one per side. The key to this move is keeping it slow and smooth. If you wish to add a challenge as you gain confidence with this move, you can lift your upper leg straight up as high as you can, so that your lower half makes an "X". If you want to add another challenge, add a push-up each time you return to the starting point.

Side Shuffle

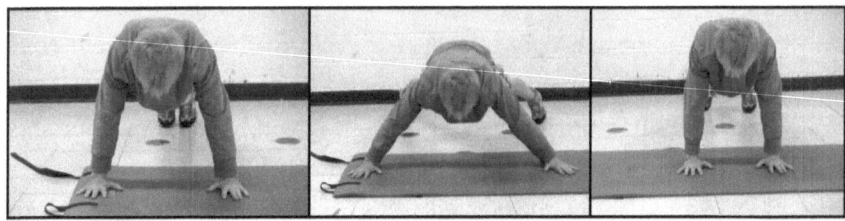

From the starting point, move to one side by shuffling one leg (let's say start on the left side as an example) over as far as you can. Then move/slide your left hand over as far as possible. The half way point here should look similar to your body making an "X" on the ground. Keep in mind though, that the only part of you that is allowed to touch the ground during this exercise are your hands and feet. Once you reach this X point, slide your right hand towards your left hand to bring you into the starting position, then your right foot back towards your left. Now repeat that move on the opposite side. As you begin, don't get disappointed if you can't get completely stretched out and make that perfect X. You know what to shoot for, though, as time goes on.

Inch Worm

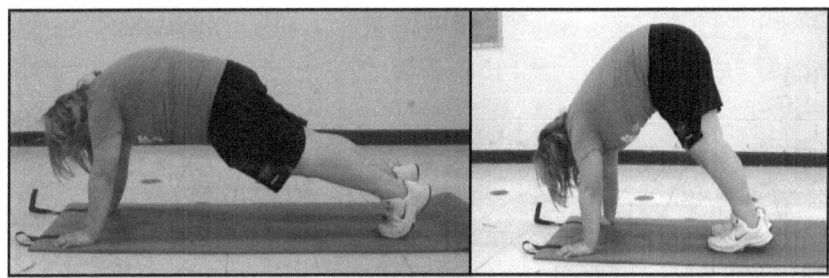

This is one of my personal favorites. From the starting point, walk your feet up toward your hands as close as you can, but keep your legs straight (you will basically be taking baby steps). When you can't go any further, walk your hands away from your feet (as with the feet, keep your hand movement to short distances). As you walk your hands out, make sure your arms stay straight. Once you have returned to the starting point, walk your hands to your feet, and then walk your feet away from your hands. You will wind up walking one forward and one backward. The only part of you that should be bending is your hips. Make sure the upper and lower half stay straight as you move them. The rep count for this is a little different, as one forward would be one, and adding the one backward would be two, and so forth.

Chair Dip

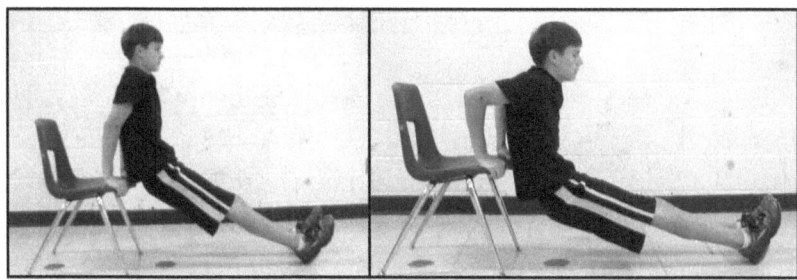

For this move, you will need a special tool (a chair). As you begin this exercise, keep your back as close to the chair without scraping. Allowing your body to get too far away will put undue pressure on your joints. Start with your legs straight, arms locked. Slowly bend your elbows to 90 degrees and return to the straight arm position. Work to keep your elbows close to your body as you go down (do not let them flare out). As you begin, you may wish to keep your knees bent and your feet closer to being under your butt. This will help you build the proper form if you cannot keep your legs straight. If you wish to challenge yourself, you could (once you get comfortable and are able to keep your legs straight) raise one leg, and switch legs every 5 repetitions. If you want even more of a challenge, put your feet up on a chair also (you can also do the raise one leg from the two chair move, if you want to super duper challenge yourself down the road).

Whacky Jack

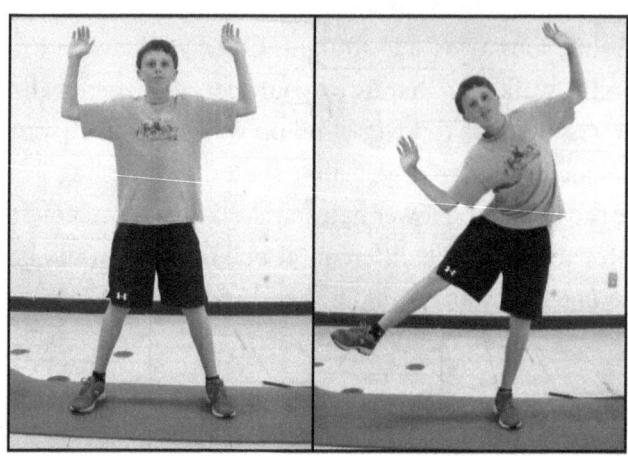

This is a very fun exercise, and also one of my favorites. It is somewhat similar to a jumping jack. The difference here is, keep your elbows bent at 90 degrees, and you kick to the side, one leg at a time. Keep your legs straight, and drive your elbows towards your hips. It may take a little time to develop this, but keep working. In the beginning, you can move slowly to develop the form, but, as time goes by, work to move as quickly as you can while maintaining the proper side-kick leg movement. A rep for this would be one on each side equals one. I usually count a rep for each time my left leg hits the floor.

Twist Wrist Push-up

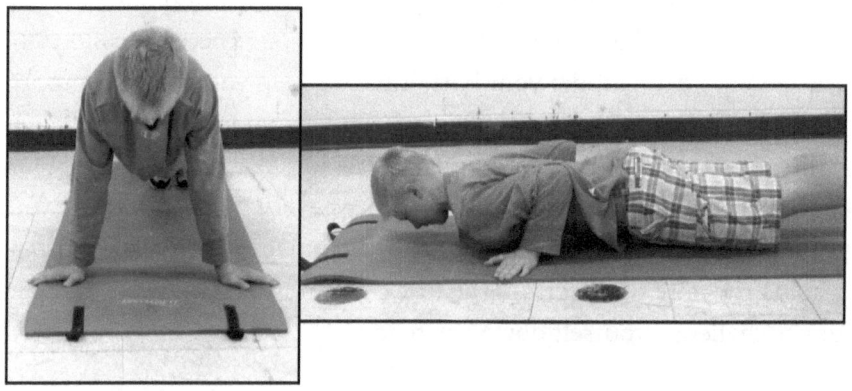

Everything as far as body position is the same as the starting point in a traditional push up. The difference with your hands is that (as the picture shows) your wrists are turned somewhere around 90 degrees so that your fingers are pointing outward. As you do this, you won't be able to keep your hands under your shoulders. They should line up more toward the bottom of your rib cage. If this feels like it may tweak your wrists, turn them to less than 90 degrees, but keep them down at the bottom of your ribs. The rest of your body should remain in the starting point as you move. If, as time goes by, you want to challenge yourself (not that this move isn't a challenge in itself), you can raise one leg and switch legs every 5 reps. For this one, leave the push-up bars (if you are using them) out.

Incline Push-up (push-up bars)

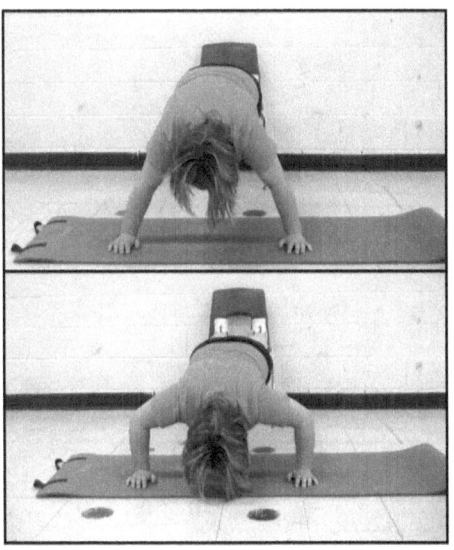

For this move you will need the chair again. Place your feet on the chair, and get on your tip toes. From this angle, maintain that straightness of the starting point, and do as many perfect push-ups as you can. As you get started with this program, if putting your feet on the chair is too difficult, you could turn the chair sideways so you can slide more of your leg onto the chair.

Dive Bomber (push-up bars)

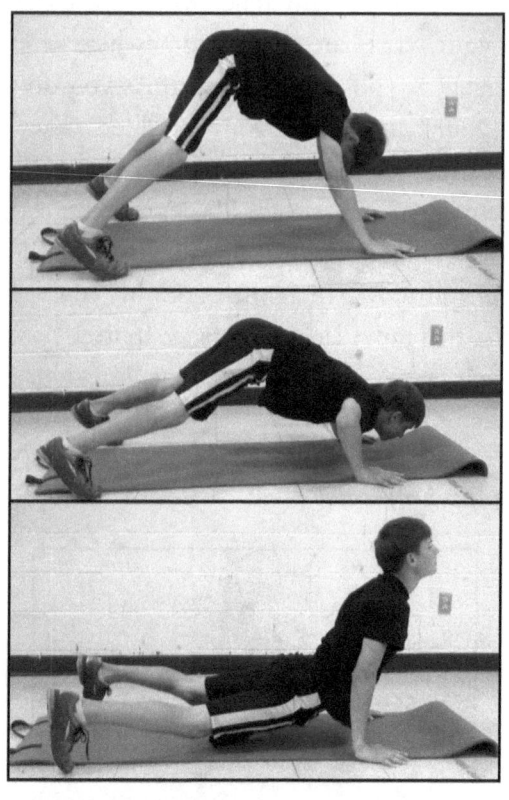

Start this move in a position similar to the A-frame Push-up, but not as much angle. Your hands should be out in front or your head and body. Also, as you can see from the picture, you are to keep your feet wide for this exercise. This is sort of a 3-stage move. The first part is to lower your face toward the ground. As you get close to touching your face to the floor, slide your body slightly forward, as if you were going to hit your chest to the floor. Continue moving forward as if you were getting into the cobra stretch, but do not allow your hips to touch the ground. To return to the start, move back in reverse order. Keep this move as smooth as possible. Think of this movement like this: head, chest, hips, hips, chest, and head. In the beginning, it may be difficult to go both forward and back. You can modify this move by going through the forward movements and when you get to your hips above the ground, push your arms straight and bend up to the starting position at the waist.

Horizontal Pull-up (push-up bars)

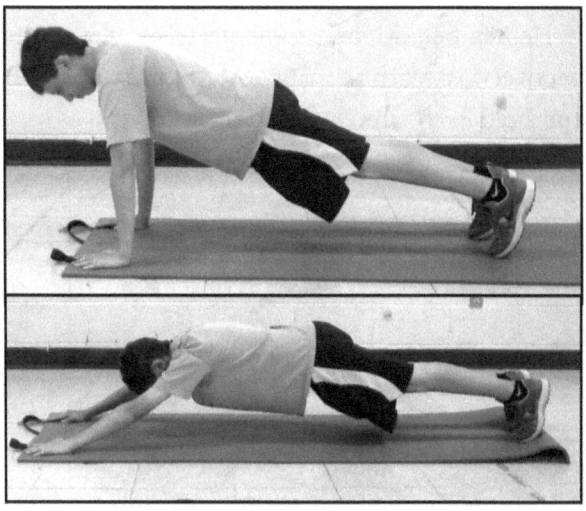

From the starting point, walk your feet backwards as far as you can, while keeping your entire body from your wrists to your calves as straight as possible. If you are really good, you will sort of look like Super Man as you get to the half way point (if you don't get there right away, then the goal is to look like that). As with the Side Shuffle, the only parts of you touching the floor should be your hands and feet. From this position, pull yourself forward. This is tough, and you may not be able to do more than a couple as you begin this program, but keep working. As you pull, you will also need to tip toe your feet back into the starting point. Be *very* conscious of your doing more pull than walking. It might take a few workouts to get this move down, but keep at it. You will know when you are doing it right when you feel it through your abdominal region as well as in your Lateralis muscles (along the side of your ribs).

Lower Body Stretches

Before we get into the workout, we can't forget the warm up and stretch. I will assume that you took a couple of minutes to do your running in place and/or jumping jacks to get the muscles ready for a good stretch. Remember, do these same stretches when you are finished to aid with recovery. As with the Upper/Abs stretches, go through each 2-3 times, and hold each stretch for 10-30 seconds.

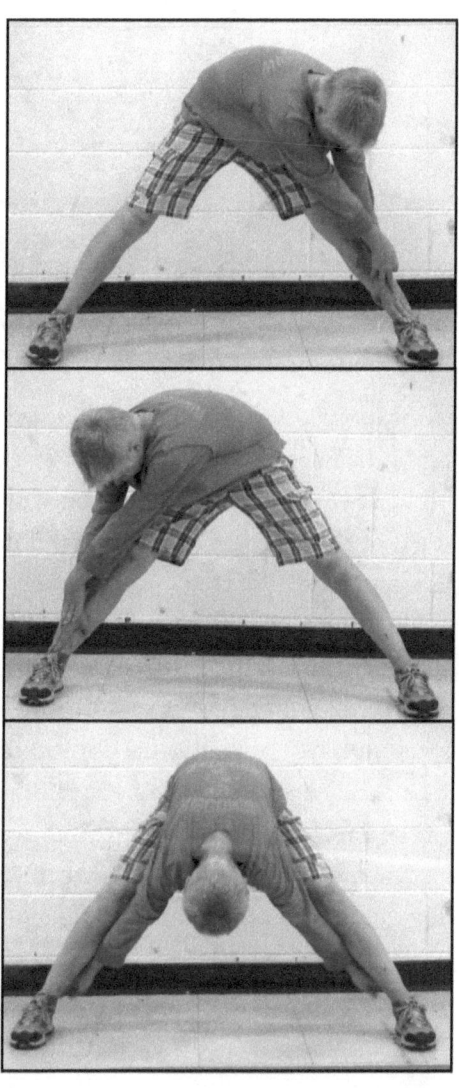

Stand with your feet wide apart, toes pointing forward. Lean to your left, trying to touch your chest to your knee. Hold your leg locked, and do not allow your knee to bend. If you can't reach your knee, stretch as far as you can and hold it. Lean to the right in the same manner. To finish, lean forward, and grab the back of your ankles, if possible. If you can't reach your ankles, reach down as far as you can towards your feet. If this is easy, reach inside your legs and grab your heels. If this still isn't enough stretch, then reach between your feet as far back as you can. (Hamstring Stretch)

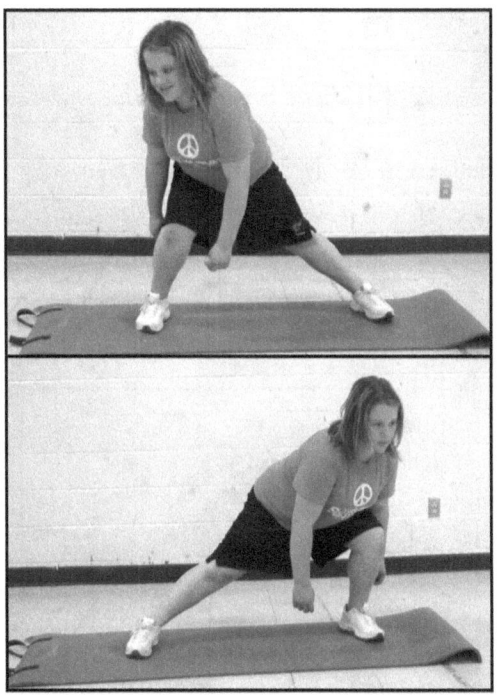

In the same position as above, keep your left leg straight and your left foot on the ground. Bend your right knee and lean to the right as far as possible and hold. Repeat this on the other side. (Groin Stretch)

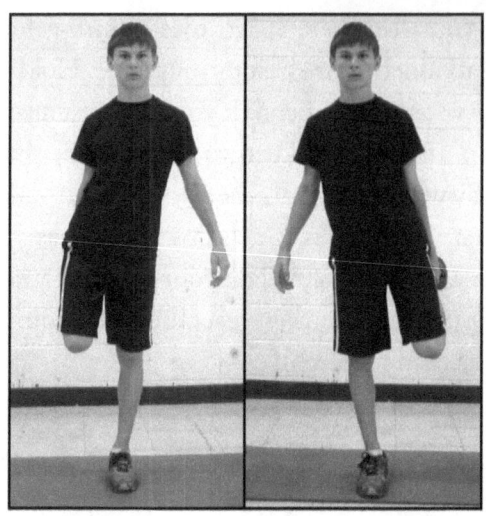

Stand tall, feet shoulder width apart, grab one leg (you may need help with balance, so use a wall, stool, or whatever) and pull the sole of your shoe up toward your butt. Make sure to stand up tall, and keep your bent knee aiming toward the floor and not off to the side. (Standing Quad Stretch)

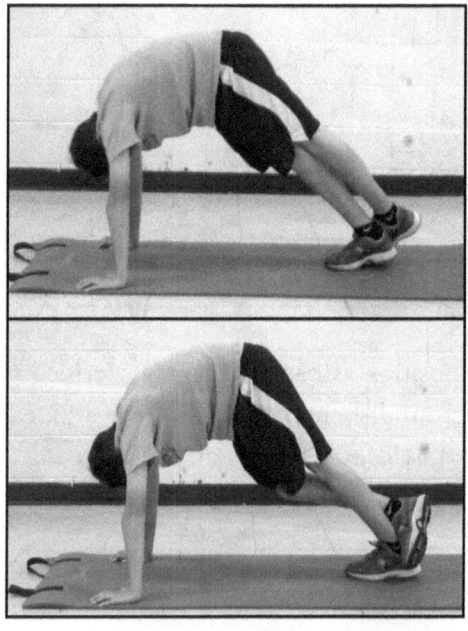

With your hands and feet on the ground and your butt in the air, place your left foot on top of your right foot (right foot should stay flat on the ground). If you don't feel this stretch in your calf, ark your backside higher in the air. Switch feet so that you have the right foot over the left and repeat. (Calf Stretch)

Lower Body Workout

Many of these moves are designed not only to strengthen your legs, but will challenge your balance, as well. I meant it to be that way. Should you stumble and fall, that's ok. Keep working. Over time you will get better. The starting point position for this one (for the most part) will be head forward, back straight, slight bend in the knees, and feet shoulder width apart. If the starting point varies from this, I will explain as we go. For the squat-type moves, do not allow your knees to go farther than a 90 degree angle. As with the Upper/Abs, you can work to a specific number, work for the time (1-minute max), or use a hybrid combination of both. You decide what is best for you.

Hindu Squat

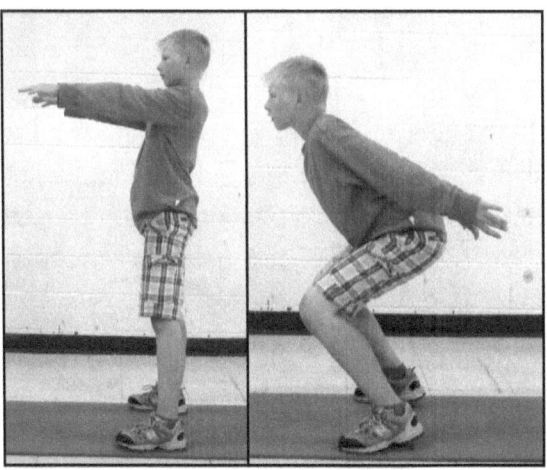

From the starting point, raise your arms so that they are straight out in front of you (this will help with balance as you move). Keep your back straight as you bend at the knees and lower yourself to that 90 degree angle in the knee. As you lower yourself, get up on your tip toes and allow your arms to drop down behind you. Hold for a second, and then return to the starting point with your arms out in front of you.

1-Leg Deadlift

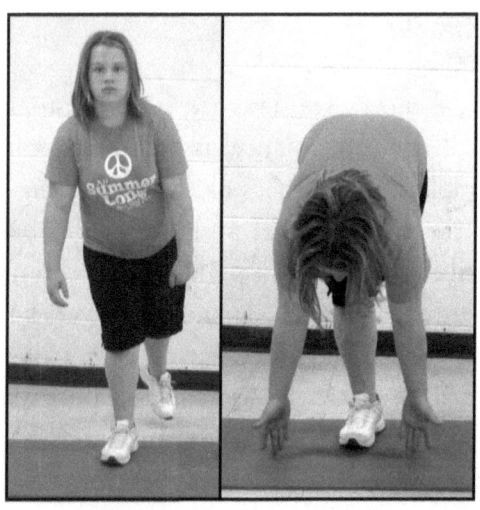

From the starting point, lean forward, while raising one leg straight out behind you. As you lean, you will naturally have to bend your knee. Keep this bend minimal. You should feel this move in your hamstrings and butt (back of your leg), not in your quadriceps (front of your leg). If you can, touch the floor in front of you with both hands. This move is to be done slowly. Once you have touched the floor (or gotten as low as you can get), return to the starting position. I recommend that you work one leg fully before working the other (go 30 seconds per leg). Notice, also, that as you lean forward, you keep your head in that neutral, looking ahead position. There is a tendency to want to look straight out in front of you, which can put unneeded stress on the neck. Think of is as looking at the wall, and leaning at the hips to look at the floor. Upon returning to the upright position, it is ok to tap your leg on the floor to help maintain your balance. As you reach towards the ground, keep your palms facing forward.

Back Bends

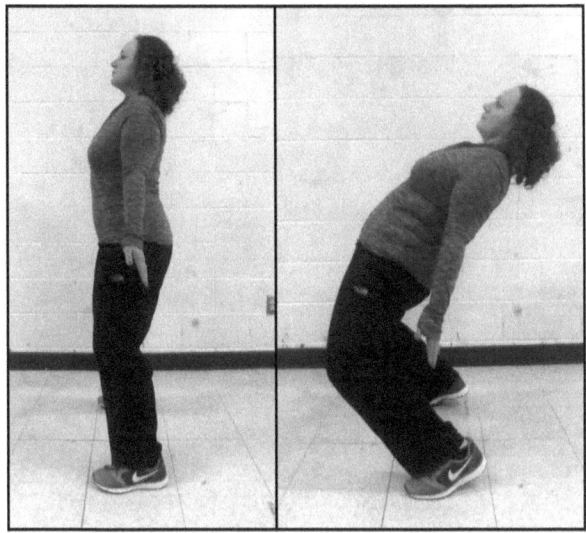

You may need to widen your feet a little bit on this one to help with balance (maybe ½ a step). From this slightly varied starting point, bend your knees and reach your arms behind you, as if you are trying to grab your ankles. As you lean back, raise up to your tip toes. This may take a bit to get used to, but stick with it. If you stumble, reset yourself and keep going. You may find it easier to allow your chin to touch your chest as you lean back, and that is ok. What you do not want to do is allow your head to sort of flop backwards and look behind you. This will throw off your balance. Lastly, as you reach for your heels, keep your palms facing forward.

Flutter Kicks

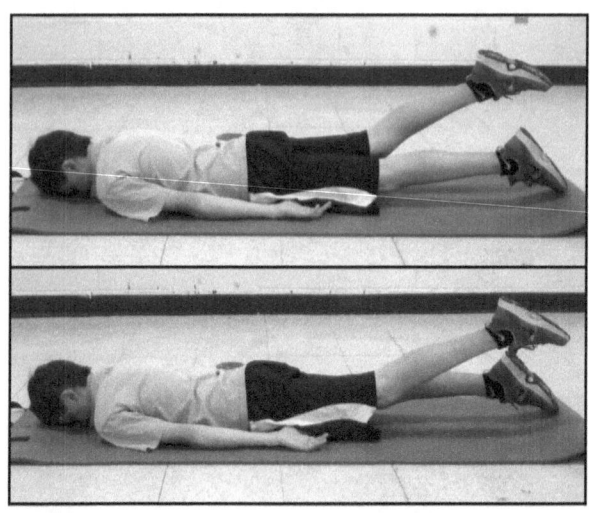

Unless you are working out on a carpeted surface, a mat is much recommended for this move. Lay as flat as possible on your stomach. Notice in the picture that as much as possible you keep your head in the neutral position (rest your forehead on the mat). It is much more comfortable to let your arms rest at your sides, palms up. An easy way to count reps for this move would be to start by raising your right leg and lowering your left. Then each time your left leg is in the low position, you count a rep. Keep your knees locked and legs as straight as possible for this exercise. Once you start, work to keep your legs off the ground during the entire move. Start with your legs at the same level (as much of your legs off the ground as possible), then raise one leg at a time as high as you can and return it to the level before raising the other leg. Make sure your toes stay pointed away from you the entire move. Ideally, the only joint that should be moving is the hip. If you feel this in your lower back to the back of your knee, you are doing it right.

Wall Sits

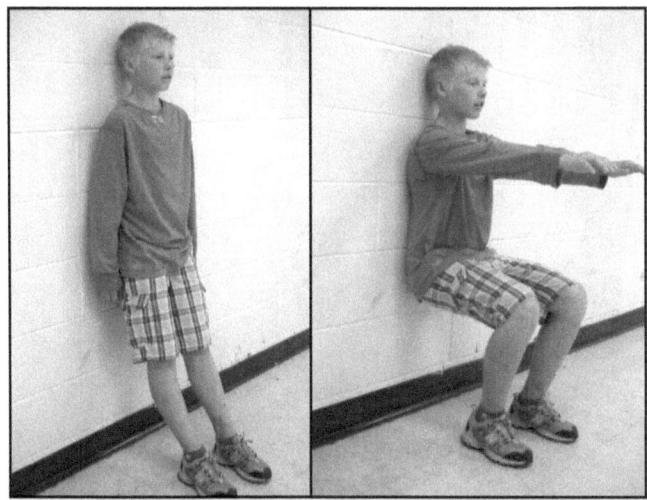

For this move you will have to go for a set time. Begin with your feet shoulder width apart, about 12-16 inches off of the wall (farther if you are longer legged, closer if you have shorter legs). Keeping your upper body straight, lean your entire back against the wall, including the back of your head. Squat down until your knees are at the 90 degree mark, and raise your arms out so that they are parallel to the ground (if this is too hard in the beginning, you can lay your palms along the wall as you squat down). If you have never done these before, I will let you know that they are very difficult. It may be something you have to work up to, and that's ok. If you need to, you can take active rests by raising your body up slightly for a few moments to decrease the angle in your knees. As time goes by, if you want more of a challenge, you can raise one leg for a few moments, and then the other.

Tip Toe Leaners

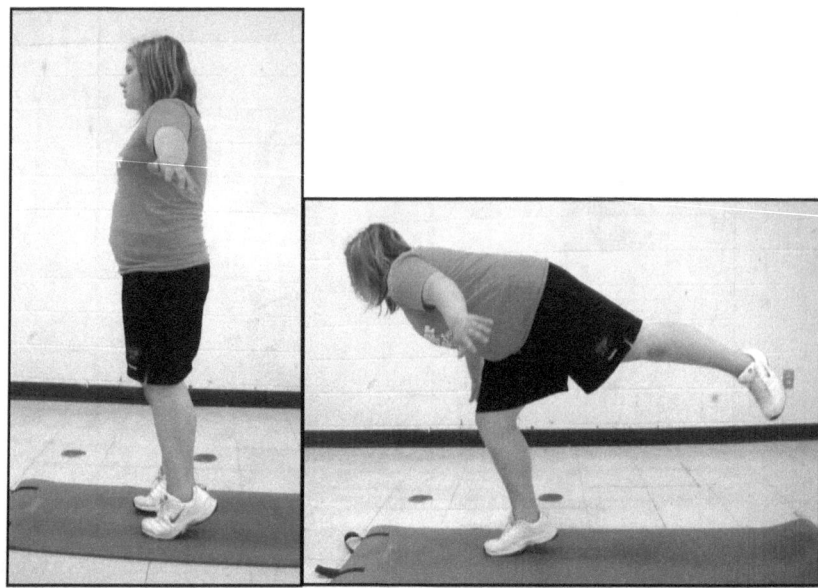

From the starting point, get up on the tip toes of one foot, and raise the other leg. Extend your arms out to the side, and lean forward until you are at a 90 degree angle in your hips. As you lean forward, maintain the neutral head position with a straight back. I think of it as using the hip joint to switch from looking at the wall to looking at the floor. Return to the starting point and repeat on the other leg. As you can imagine, working both legs equals 1 rep. You may find that at first, you can't get to the 90 degree point without stumbling a bit. You will get there. Lean as far forward as you can, and then return. Also, you may find that it is easier on one side than the other. Keep working, you will improve over time. Another reminder is that this should be done as a steady, slow move. Speed here will have you falling all over and getting nothing from this.

Plyo-Jump

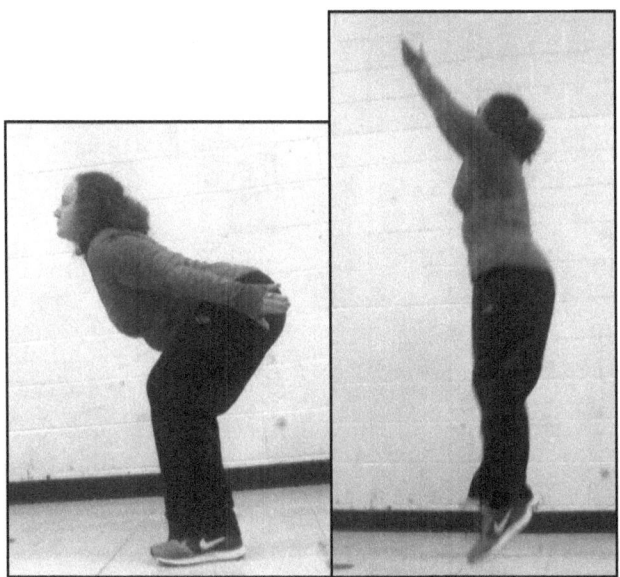

The starting point for this is very much like the half way point of the Hindu Squat. The only real difference is that while you are bent your feet are flat on the ground. From this starting position, jump as high as you can, straight up in the air, and throw your arms over your head. When you land, land on your toes. I want to stress this: *land on your toes!* It is very important and also a safety factor. Keep your landings as quiet as possible. Landing on your toes will allow you to cushion the landing a lot more than landing heels first or flat footed. As you land, recoil yourself into the starting position. Make sure you come to a *complete stop* before jumping again. Each jump should be its own, one rep explosive move. Some people form a bad habit of doing this move continually like a jack rabbit. There should be a distinct, although short, pause between each jump. Make each one perfect. For me, it helps to count the rep as I come to the recoil position. This assures that I come to a complete stop between jumps.

Sneaky Lunge

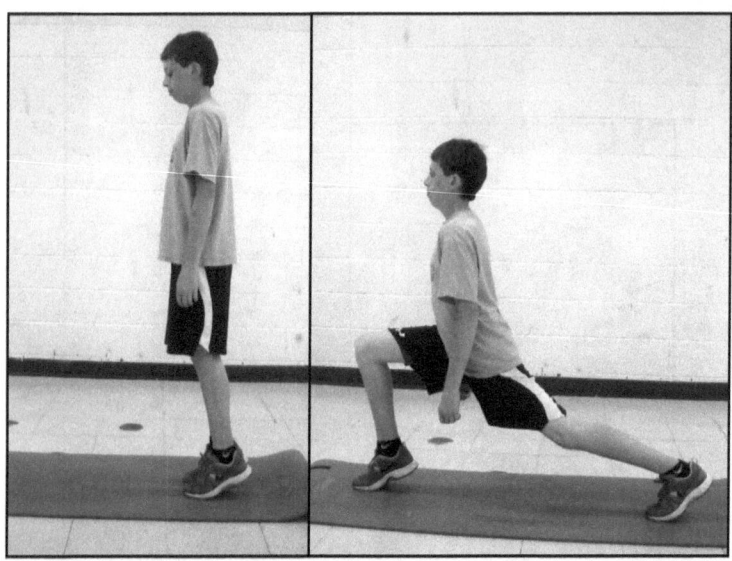

This whole exercise is done on your tip toes, hence the name the Sneaky Lunge. From the starting point, rise up to your tip toes. One leg at a time, take a slightly exaggerated step out in front of you (somewhere in the approximate range of 36-40 inches). If you have really long legs, your step will obviously need to be longer. As you step out, keep your back leg straight. Once your front foot hits the ground, bend your knee to 90 degrees, and lean forward just enough so that the bottom of your ribs touch your thigh. From this position, explode up and bring your foot back to the starting position. Repeat on the other side. As you step out and begin to lean, you may find that you need to put your arms out for balance, which is fine. If you are really good (or if you want a goal to strive for), keep your arms at your sides as you step out and lean. One repetition equals one lunge per leg.

Alternating Knee Bends

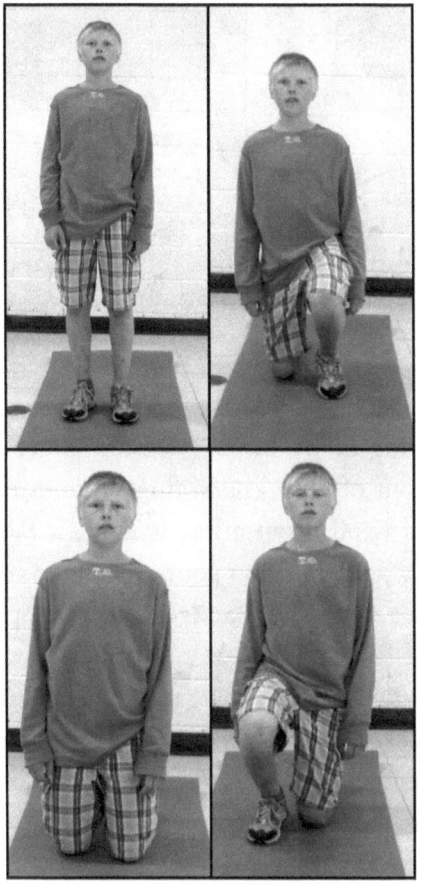

For this, I recommend that you stand on a mat to help protect your knees. From the starting point, lower yourself to the ground, one knee at a time. Once both knees are on the ground, raise yourself up, one knee at a time, to the starting point. This can get confusing, so think of a movement pattern something like this as you go through this exercise: right knee down, left knee down, right knee up, left knee up. Then for the next rep, left knee down, right knee down, left knee up, right knee up.

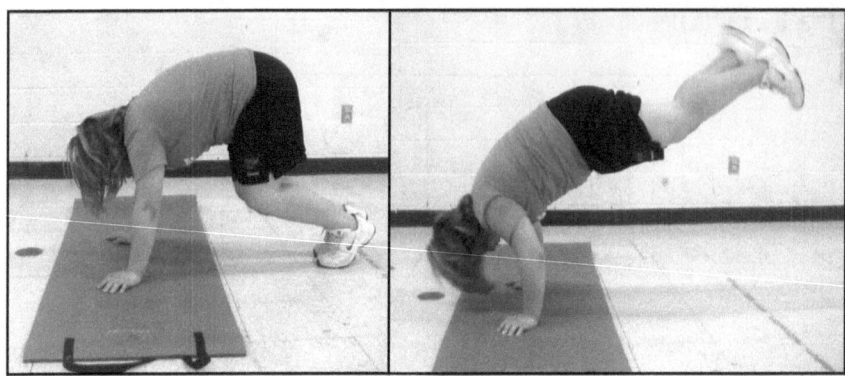

Mule Kick

From the starting point, bend down and place your hands about 16-18 inches in front of your knees, fingers pointing away from you. Your hands should wind up in a line with your face, just to the side of your head. From here, position yourself so that your body weight is evenly distributed between your hands and feet. Keep your hands firmly placed on the floor (a mat would help for both comfort and traction). Once you achieve this position, drive your legs up and away from your body as far out and straight as you can (like a mule would if it kicked). While in the air, recoil your knees so that you land softly on your toes. Like the Plyo-Jump, come to a complete stop before each rep.

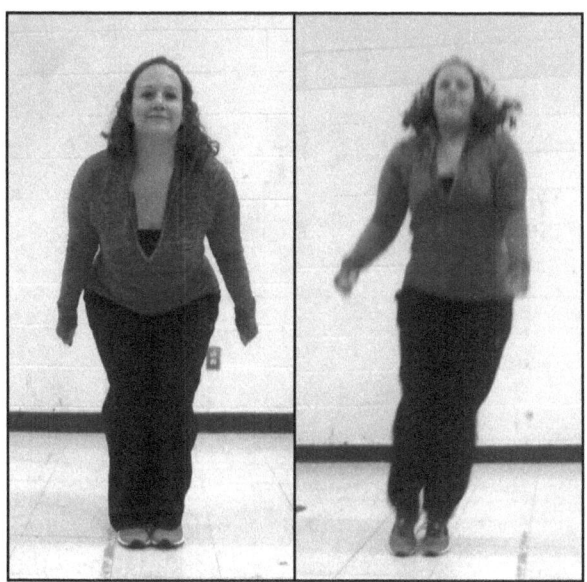

Side Hops

For this move, it may help to have a soft target such as a towel to jump over. For your own sake, do not use anything that will possibly cause injury if you land on it (like a water bottle). It seems almost silly to mention that, but I have been around a while and have seen people do some silly things when it comes to exercise. This is a simple move. You can do this a few ways. The ultimate move would be to jump, knees bent, side to side, over a towel (or a spot on the floor), keeping your distance from start to landing about 12 inches. Jump with your knees slightly bent, and land softly on your toes. If, in the beginning, this is too much (as it is near the end of the work out, and your legs by this point should be feeling fairly spent), you could step, one foot at a time over, or, straighten your legs and pounce over using your calf muscles (should you choose this, you should still land on your toes and cushion your landing by slightly bending your knees). Unlike the Mule Kick or Plyo-Jump, this move is for speed, so each time you hit the ground leap back over like a rabbit. One repetition equals one hop over and then back.

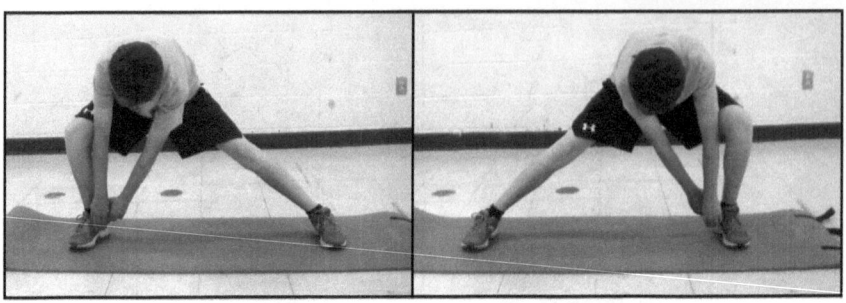

Wide Leg Side-Side Leans

Begin with your feet as wide apart as when you warmed up and did the Hamstring Stretch. From this position, bend one knee, while keeping the other leg straight and both feet flat on the floor. From here, s-l-o-w-l-y move to the other direction, bending the other knee and straightening your leg. During this move, keep your finger tips softly touching the ground as you move from side to side. If, in the beginning, it is too difficult to keep your fingers on the ground (or if you feel a little funny in your lower back), bring your hands up and grab hold of your hips, but be conscious of keeping your butt low and in the same plane as you move from side to side. Over time, work to be able to gently let your fingers drag on the ground as you move. As you move (let's say to the left), you want to slide your body across far enough so that your right hand winds up in front of your left foot . Obviously, reverse that when moving to the right.

Conclusion

- -

As you finish reading, I want to leave you with a few things to think about. First, don't be afraid to re-read certain sections of this book. I know that, for myself, I may have "read" something, but I don't always get everything out of it the first time through. If you can't remember something, or have questions, pull it off the shelf and re-reference what you are looking for, especially as you get started.

Second, I cannot stress enough that fitness is a 3-pronged attack. Exercise, diet, and rest are all key components for complete fitness. If you short yourself in one area, you are hurting all three. Forming good habits is not easy, but it is worthwhile.

You may find that, over time, doing these same moves in the same order can become a bit old or stale. It is not uncommon to sort of build up a tolerance to a routine. If you find yourself in this position, don't lose your motivation! Once you have the routine and moves down pat, if you feel like you are possibly losing interest in the order of this routine, then start at another point. Many times, just changing the order will be plenty to keep you motivated. For at least the first 6 weeks, though, go at it in the order it is written, to make sure you have it down solid. Also, if you do choose a different point to begin, follow along in that order, to keep a balanced attack as you work out.

Lastly, you spent the money to buy this book, and took the time to read it. That's a great start. Now is the time for the real decision. Are you going to stick with it? Are you going to discipline yourself to make this routine part of your day? Are you going to work through the initial pain and continue? Are you going to (if needed) change your eating habits to make your workout that much more beneficial? These are questions only you can answer. I hope that your answer is yes to all of them, for your sake. Start now. Don't wait for that time when you are feeling motivated, or put it off and start on the next Monday, or whatever day you choose so you can keep up with the whole routine, start now. The sooner you begin the sooner you will be rewarded with the benefits of better health.

So there you have it. Before you get to working out, I want to thank you for taking your time to read this and spending your money to purchase this book. I truly appreciate it. Keep at it. If this is your first time exercising, keep in mind that we all start somewhere. If you have worked out before, welcome yourself to a new challenge. If you haven't worked out in a while but are getting back into it, you have made a good choice.

I view exercise as a competition, but not like X's versus O's or Home versus Away. I see it as you versus you. Whatever anyone else is doing should not matter. This is about you getting in shape, living healthy, and kicking some butt. This is about you gaining confidence. This is about you disciplining yourself to become better. The bottom line is, this is about you. Don't quit!

Appendix

I have included for you a sheet that should be easy for you to photocopy and help you track your workouts. I encourage you to fill them out in full every time you workout, and save them. One thing (I hope) you will find is setting a daily goal helps keep you focused on a weekly goal. Hitting a weekly goal will help you stay focused on that long term goal you have. Also, as time goes on, see where you started and where you are now. Sometimes, it is hard to see the progress when you are in the middle of working, and anyone could get frustrated and want to give up. Look at how you have progressed! Keep going!

"NO EXCUSES"   My goal this week is: _____

WORKOUT WORKSHEET

UPPER/ABS	Goal: MONDAY	Goal: TUESDAY	Goal: WEDNESDAY	Goal: THURSDAY	Goal: FRIDAY
DATE:					
1. 3-Stage Push-up	/ / /	/ / /	/ / /	/ / /	/ / /
2. Horizontal Side Knee Lift	/ / /	/ / /	/ / /	/ / /	/ / /
3. A-Frame Push-up	/ / /	/ / /	/ / /	/ / /	/ / /
4. Side-Side Plank	/ / /	/ / /	/ / /	/ / /	/ / /
5. Side Shuffle	/ / /	/ / /	/ / /	/ / /	/ / /
6. Inch Worm	/ / /	/ / /	/ / /	/ / /	/ / /
7. Chair Dip	/ / /	/ / /	/ / /	/ / /	/ / /
8. Whacky Jack	/ / /	/ / /	/ / /	/ / /	/ / /
9. Twist Wrist Push-up	/ / /	/ / /	/ / /	/ / /	/ / /
10. Decline up Push-up	/ / /	/ / /	/ / /	/ / /	/ / /
11. Dive Bomber	/ / /	/ / /	/ / /	/ / /	/ / /
12. Horizontal Pull-up	/ / /	/ / /	/ / /	/ / /	/ / /

LOWER	Goal: MONDAY	Goal: TUESDAY	Goal: WEDNESDAY	Goal: THURSDAY	Goal: FRIDAY
DATE:					
1. Hindu Squat	/ / /	/ / /	/ / /	/ / /	/ / /
2. 1-Leg Deadlift	/ / /	/ / /	/ / /	/ / /	/ / /
3. Back Bends	/ / /	/ / /	/ / /	/ / /	/ / /
4. Flutter Kicks	/ / /	/ / /	/ / /	/ / /	/ / /
5. Wall Sits	/ / /	/ / /	/ / /	/ / /	/ / /
6. Tip Toe Leaners	/ / /	/ / /	/ / /	/ / /	/ / /
7. Plyo-Jump	/ / /	/ / /	/ / /	/ / /	/ / /
8. Sneaky Lunge	/ / /	/ / /	/ / /	/ / /	/ / /
9. Alternating Knee Bends	/ / /	/ / /	/ / /	/ / /	/ / /
10. Mule Kick	/ / /	/ / /	/ / /	/ / /	/ / /
11. Side Hops	/ / /	/ / /	/ / /	/ / /	/ / /
12. Wide Leg Side-Side Leans	/ / /	/ / /	/ / /	/ / /	/ / /

50

Author Biography

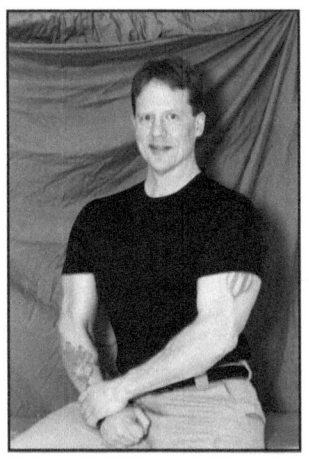

For the past thirty plus years, Jeff Hauswirth has been involved with fitness in some form or fashion, whether as an athlete, a coach, a teacher or a trainer. During his years in the military, while serving in the United States Navy as a Hospital Corpsman, and Combat Medic, Jeff created many exercise programs for his fellow shipmates. Currently, Jeff teaches Physical Education and Health at the same school that he graduated from. Jeff helps get younger kids on the path to health and fitness by running the school weight room and cardio area. Jeff is also a certified American Council on Exercise (A.C.E.) Health Coach, and has worked with many people of all ages in not only fitness program development, but dietary education as well as behavioral changes. Jeff has coached football, hockey, and track. He currently lives in Michigan with his wife and three children